Senior Executive Transportation & Public Safety Summit

June 26 - 27, 2012
Washington, DC

National Traffic Incident Management Leadership & Innovation
Roadmap for Success

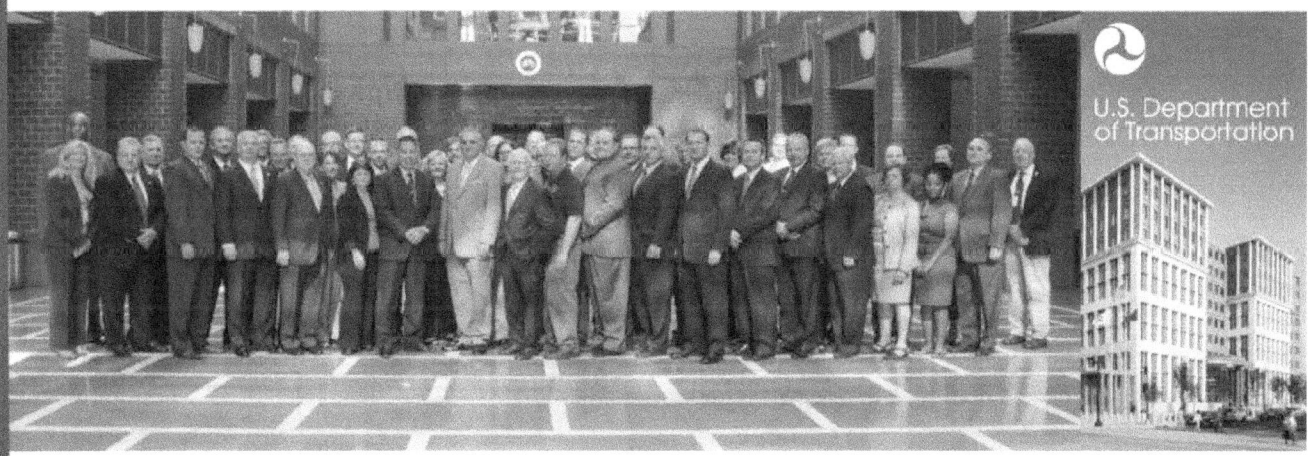

**U.S. Department
of Transportation**

TRANSPORTATION
AND PUBLIC SAFETY

1. Report No. FHWA-HOP-12-051	2. Government Accession No.	3. Recipient's Catalog No.	
4. Title and Subtitle *Senior Executive Transportation & Public Safety Summit: National Traffic Incident Management Leadership & Innovation Roadmap for Success*		5. Report Date 09-05-12	
		6. Performing Organization Code HOTO	
7. Author(s) Cassandra Allwell, David Perlman and Luisa Paiewonsky, Volpe & Kimberly C. Vásconez and Tim Lane, FHWA Office of Transportation Operations		8. Performing Organization Report No.	
9. Performing Organization Name and Address John A. Volpe National Transportation Systems Center U.S. DOT/Research and Innovative Technology Administration 55 Broadway Cambridge, MA 02142-1093		10. Work Unit No. (TRAIS) TI&EM	
		11. Contract or Grant No.	
12. Sponsoring Agency Name and Address Federal Highway Administration Office of Operations 1200 New Jersey Avenue, SE, Washington, DC 20590		13. Type of Report and Period Covered Meeting Proceedings; 06-26 & 27-2012	
		14. Sponsoring Agency Code FHWA-HOTO	
15. Supplementary Notes Tim Lane, Public Safety Program Manager, Traffic Incident & Events Management, HOTO/HOP/FHWA as Government Task Monitor and Event Organizer			

16. Abstract

This report summarizes the proceedings, findings, and recommendations from a two-day Senior Executive Summit on Transportation and Public Safety, held June 26 and 27, 2012 at the United States Department of Transportation (USDOT) in Washington, D.C. This forum of senior-level, multi-disciplinary executives representing the transportation, law enforcement, fire and rescue, and emergency medical services communities addressed major challenges and innovative solutions in enhancing the state of the practice nationally in Traffic Incident Management (TIM). Secretary of Transportation Ray LaHood, Federal Highway Administration (FHWA) Deputy Administrator Greg Nadeau, and FHWA Executive Director Jeff Paniati provided opening remarks expressing the commitment of the entire Department to support safe, quick traffic incident response on the Nation's roadways. Participants at the Summit discussed innovative practices in TIM policies, legislation, training and outreach. Summit highlights included discussions and presentations on the following issues: Improving responder and motorist safety and consistency among jurisdictions; Supporting TIM outreach initiatives and messaging; Enhancing State and local legislation and policies that advance TIM planning and operations, including Driver Removal and Authority Removal legislation; Supporting urgent and clearly-defined research strategies, such as model Move Over and Driver Removal laws, the effects of emergency lighting, and the impact of TIM performance measures; Implementing the National TIM Responder Training course developed through the Transportation Research Board's Second Strategic Highway Research Program (SHRP 2); Improving the efficiency of the highway system through possible cost-recovery strategies, better investment of cost-efficient resources, and improved communication among responders about roles and responsibilities; and Developing an action-based executive group equipped to provide leadership, support, and guidance in advancing priority actions.

17. Key Words Traffic Incident Management; Safety; Law Enforcement; Public Safety; Congestion		18. Distribution Statement No restrictions on distribution to the public	
19. Security Classif. (of this report) Unclassified	20. Security Classif. (of this page) Unclassified	21. No. of Pages 36	22. Price $0

(Page Intentionally Left Blank)

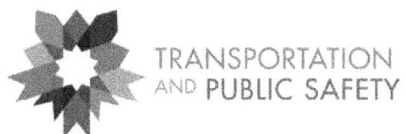

TRANSPORTATION AND PUBLIC SAFETY

Executive Summary

This report summarizes the proceedings, findings, and recommendations from a two-day Senior Executive Summit on Transportation and Public Safety, held June 26 and 27, 2012 at the United States Department of Transportation (USDOT) in Washington, D.C. This forum of senior-level, multi-disciplinary executives representing the transportation, law enforcement, fire and rescue, and emergency medical services communities addressed major challenges and innovative solutions in enhancing the state of the practice nationally in Traffic Incident Management (TIM). Secretary of Transportation Ray LaHood, Federal Highway Administration (FHWA) Deputy Administrator Greg Nadeau, and FHWA Executive Director Jeff Paniati provided opening remarks expressing the commitment of the entire Department to support safe, quick traffic incident response on the Nation's roadways.

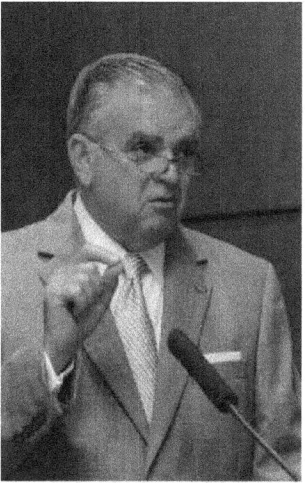

Figure 1: Secretary of Transportation Ray LaHood addresses leaders in the fields of public safety and transportation on June 26, 2012

Participants at the Summit discussed innovative practices in TIM policies, legislation, training and outreach. Summit highlights included discussions and presentations on the following issues:

- Improving responder and motorist safety and consistency among jurisdictions;
- Supporting TIM outreach initiatives and messaging;
- Enhancing State and local legislation and policies that advance TIM planning and operations, including Driver Removal and Authority Removal legislation;
- Supporting urgent and clearly-defined research strategies, such as model Move Over and Driver Removal laws, the effects of emergency lighting, and the impact of TIM performance measures;
- Implementing the National TIM Responder Training course developed through the Transportation Research Board's Second Strategic Highway Research Program (SHRP 2);
- Improving the efficiency of the highway system through possible cost-recovery strategies, better investment of cost-efficient resources, and improved communication among responders about roles and responsibilities; and
- Developing an action-based executive group equipped to provide leadership, support, and guidance in advancing priority actions.

Through presentations and group discussions, Summit participants identified challenges, opportunities, and recommendations. Notable challenges included institutionalization and sustainability of TIM practices, consistency between States in TIM legislation, public awareness regarding TIM laws and policies, and understanding among responder groups of both discipline-specific and shared priorities and goals. Participants identified regular and frequent communication between responder groups, increased measurement of incident and roadway

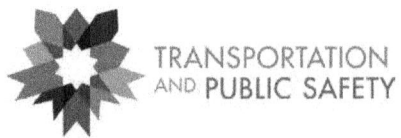

TRANSPORTATION AND PUBLIC SAFETY

clearance times and secondary crashes, and enhanced public outreach and training campaigns as significant opportunities to address these pressing challenges. Participants also proposed the following recommendations for FHWA's consideration:

- **Establish a small, executive-level working group with membership from the key organizations that represent TIM practitioners.** This group should meet up to twice per year to discuss TIM issues of national significance and identify barriers to, and opportunities to promote, progress towards national goals. A Technical Working Group should also be formed to act in a consultative capacity to the Executive Working Group and a National Networking Group should provide a forum for TIM practitioners to share information on the state of the practice.

- **Deploy National TIM Responder Training** through USDOT leadership endorsement and State-level transportation and public safety summits and executive briefings. Training attendance should be promoted based on the intended training outcomes – improved responder safety, rapid treatment of crash victims, and efficient incident clearance – and encouraged through the availability of continuing education credits and an online format.

- **Promote national deployment of TIM performance measures** through promotion of consistent definitions of metrics, responder education focused on the importance of performance measurement, prioritized implementation of TIM performance measures for States with limited data, and initiatives to enhance data collection. Based on participants' input, FHWA recommended the establishment of a TIM Performance Measurement Pilot.

- **Enhance consistency of, and compliance with, TIM legislation** by performing additional outreach and education for responder communities and the general public, defining model TIM legislation, and conducting additional research on practices that lead to greater compliance with laws requiring drivers to change lanes and/or reduce speed when approaching stopped emergency vehicles.

Summit participants believed that the state of the practice in TIM has never been stronger, and that national-level TIM leadership, improved communication and collaboration, a trained community of TIM practitioners, and accountability towards TIM performance targets will ultimately reduce the fatalities among emergency responders and transportation personnel.

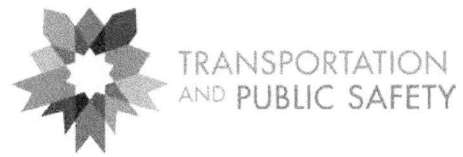

Table of Contents

EXECUTIVE SUMMARY I

I.   INTRODUCTION 1

II.   TIM STATE OF THE PRACTICE 8

III.   CHALLENGES AND OPPORTUNITIES IN ENHANCING TIM NATIONALLY 15

IV.   RECOMMENDATIONS 19

V.   VISION FOR THE FUTURE AND NEXT STEPS 27

VI.   APPENDIX A – SUMMIT PARTICIPANTS 29

VII.   APPENDIX B – SUMMIT AGENDA 32

VIII. APPENDIX C – SUMMARY OF ACTIONS 35

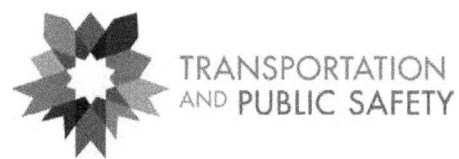
TRANSPORTATION AND PUBLIC SAFETY

I.   Introduction

Background

Recent statistics demonstrate that the Nation's roads have become safer. The year 2010 proved the safest for the Nation's roads since 1949. Nearly 25 percent fewer motor vehicle fatalities occurred in 2010 compared to the recent peak in 2005; about 40 percent fewer fatalities occurred in 2010 compared to the all-time high of the early 1970s. Moreover, vehicle travel has continually increased in that time, so the crash fatality rate has declined along with the overall number of crashes. Experts cite many reasons for the improved safety on roads. Today's vehicles include more advanced safety features while roads are designed and improved with countermeasures intended to prevent or mitigate the effects of crashes. Seat belt use has climbed, and laws addressing impaired driving have been strengthened considerably over the past several decades. Targeted enforcement and education campaigns have fostered increased awareness among drivers about the behaviors that contribute to crashes.

Nevertheless, hazards remain. Each year, dozens of emergency responders, highway workers, and tow operators are killed while responding to traffic incidents; countless more are injured or experience near-miss situations. Moving traffic threatens the safety of first responders as they provide medical assistance to victims and investigate the cause of the crash. Highway workers and tow operators are similarly at risk as they clear the scene and work to resume normal operations. Unexpected slowing, stopping, or distraction caused by the primary crash scene, represent hazards to other drivers as well.

Traffic Incident Management

Public safety and transportation agencies recognize the dangers inherent in traffic incident response. In some cases States have implemented policies and laws designed to clear roads quickly and efficiently of hazards, and to keep first responders and highway personnel safe as they work at the side of the road. Three types of general legislation constituting "Quick Clearance" laws include:

- **Move Over Laws**, which require drivers approaching a scene where emergency responders are present to either change lanes when possible and/or reduce speed;

- **Driver Removal Laws**, which require that vehicles involved in typically minor traffic incidents – with no apparent physical injury and/or minor property damage – be moved out of the travel lanes to a safe location where drivers can exchange information and/or wait for law enforcement assistance; and

- **Authority Removal Laws**, which clarify the authority and responsibility of pre-designated public agencies to clear damaged or disabled vehicles and spilled cargo from the roadway to prevent the occurrence of secondary incidents (an incident that occurs as a result of an earlier incident) and to allow normal traffic flow to resume. Authority Removal laws typically provide indemnification for these agencies if removal duties are performed in good faith and without gross negligence.

Although a number of States currently have one or more of these laws in place, observed variability in the existence, wording, and coverage of Quick Clearance laws challenges further implementation. States have also created quick clearance programs for first responder and highway personnel that include operational procedures and equipment designed to respond to

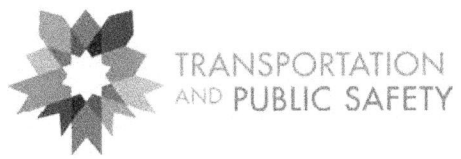

and clear an incident quickly and safely. States recognize the need for more coordinated Traffic Incident Management (TIM), creating "TIM Teams," TIM protocols, and other incident management solutions to reduce confusion and conflict at the scene and promote efficient and effective clearance.

Despite the progress made by local, regional and State transportation and public safety agencies in implementing TIM programs and procedures, effective management of crash scenes remains an elusive goal, yet an important objective of traffic incident responders. Addressing this challenge offers a great potential to improve safety for both the public and first responders. In addition to compromising safety, traffic incidents are a major cause of congestion, which wastes time, fuel, and productivity. The Texas Transportation Institute's 2011 Urban Mobility Report estimated that auto commuters in the country's 439 urban areas spent an average of 34 hours each on congested roads in 2010, amounting to nearly two billion excess gallons of consumed fuel. More efficient incident management can reduce congestion and mitigate the corresponding environmental and economic impacts.

Leadership in Transportation and Public Safety

National and Regional Organizations

A number of national-level organizations continue to achieve significant progress in advancing TIM at the national level. These organizations represent the interests of all responders and personnel involved in traffic incident management and push for further refinement of the practice to improve safety and reduce congestion. These organizations include, but are not limited to, the American Association of State Highway and Transportation Officials (AASHTO), the International Association of Chiefs of Police, (IACP), International Association of Fire Chiefs (IAFC), International Association of Fire Fighters (IAFF), National Volunteer Fire Council (NVFC), the United States Fire Administration (USFA), and the National Association of State Emergency Medical Service Officials (NASEMSO). Regional organizations like the Cumberland Valley Volunteer Firemen's Association and the I-95 Corridor Coalition promote TIM best practices by providing training resources, outreach material, and other information focused on keeping responders safe while clearing incidents quickly. Over the past decade, these groups and about 15 others coalesced under the National Traffic Incident Management Coalition (NTIMC) umbrella to provide policy and procedural guidance to the Federal Highway Administration (FHWA). As will be discussed, FHWA has assumed a leadership role in developing TIM as a new discipline within the public safety arena.

USDOT/FHWA

The United States Department of Transportation (USDOT) has made unprecedented advancements through its commitment to transportation safety, particularly on the Nation's roadways. In addition to focusing on crash prevention through anti-distracted and impaired driving initiatives, USDOT leadership has emphasized the importance of all tools that promote safety, including State and local laws (e.g. Safe, Quick Clearance), enforcement (working with inter-disciplinary groups), measurement through statistical data collection and analysis, and partnerships that focus on safety.

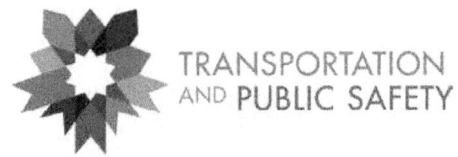

Since the 1980s, FHWA leadership has promoted TIM as an effective strategy for traffic operations, conducting research and disseminating noteworthy practices. Between 2010 and 2012, FHWA conducted TIM Advanced Practitioner Workshops for mid-level managers and outreach visits with senior decision makers – including political, law enforcement, fire and rescue, emergency medical service, metropolitan planning organization, towing, and State and local Departments of Transportation (DOTs) officials – in the country's largest 40 metropolitan areas. FHWA has used these visits to discuss the importance of TIM policies, procedures, noteworthy practices, lessons learned, performance measurement, and safe, quick clearance laws and policies.

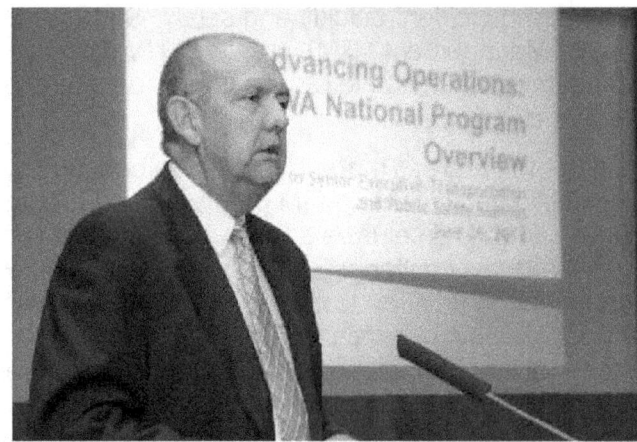

Figure 2: Jeff Lindley, FHWA Associate Administrator for Operations, discusses the agency's programs for advancing transportation operations

FHWA, with support from AASHTO and the Transportation Research Board (TRB), has also taken a leading role in deploying two products from the Second Strategic Highway Research Program (SHRP 2) that will improve traffic incident scene management. The first is a multi-disciplinary training course that promotes a shared understanding of the requirements for quick clearance and safeguards responders and drivers. The second product is a two-day "train-the-trainer" program that facilitates widespread use of the multi-disciplinary training course (more information is available in Section II). In an effort to build consensus and gain support from the public safety community on both SHRP 2 products, FHWA hosted meetings in August and December 2011 with leaders in the law enforcement and fire response communities, respectively. These meetings provided a foundation for convening leaders in all disciplines responsible for traffic incident response and safety.

National Unified Goal for Traffic Incident Management

From 2003 to 2005, FHWA, AASHTO, NTIMC, and others conducted an international scan on traffic incident response practices in Europe (for details about this scan, please see the report titled *Traffic Incident Response Practices in Europe*, published in February 2006). The findings of the group included the importance of setting a National policy that supports efforts of traffic incident responders. As a result of this significant scan, FHWA, AAHSTO, and other members of the NTIMC produced, presented, and adopted a National Unified Goal for TIM in 2007. The National Unified Goal includes a collection of 18 strategies designed to help agencies contribute to reaching the three National Unified Goal objectives (see sidebar).

The National Unified Goal serves as a National tool to be used in organizing local, regional, and State TIM programs. The adoption of the National Unified Goal was important for several reasons:

1. It formally recognized the key roles of transportation, along with traditional public safety agencies, in addressing and clearing incidents from the Nation's roadways;

2. It placed equal importance on the need for Responder Safety, Safe and Quick Clearance of Incidents, and Prompt and Reliable Communications among responders; and

3. It provided a tool in the form of 18 key strategies to be used by jurisdictions in developing health, effective TIM programs.

Today, FHWA and State and local DOTs are using the National Unified Goal to organize and enhance TIM programs in top metropolitan areas round the United States.

Senior Executive Summit on Transportation and Public Safety

Adoption of the National Unified Goal was a notable step in advancing TIM as National issue. In order to identify additional opportunities to advance the state of TIM practices, policies and programs, FHWA convened more than 50 national leaders in June 2012 in the fields of transportation, law enforcement, fire and rescue, and emergency medical services to discuss challenges and innovative solutions in promoting safe and quick response to traffic incidents. With unprecedented support for TIM from USDOT, AASHTO, and TRB through SHRP 2, as well as from IACP, IAFC, NVFC, NASEMSO, and others, FHWA anticipated that this meeting would provide an ideal opportunity to advance the state of TIM practices at the national level.

FHWA designed the executive summit to focus on:

NATIONAL UNIFIED GOAL STRATEGIES

Cross-cutting

1. *TIM Partnerships and Programs.*
2. *Multidisciplinary NIMS and TIM Training.*
3. *Goals for Performance and Progress.*
4. *TIM Technology.*
5. *Effective TIM Policies.*
6. *Awareness and Education Partnerships.*

Responder Safety

7. *Recommended Practices for Responder Safety.*
8. *Move Over/Slow Down Laws.*
9. *Driver Training and Awareness.*

Safe, Quick Clearance

10. *Multidisciplinary TIM Procedures.*
11. *Response and Clearance Time Goals.*
12. *24/7 Availability.*

Prompt, Reliable Communications

13. *Multidisciplinary Communications Practices and Procedures.*
14. *Prompt, Reliable Responder Notification.*
15. *Interoperable Voice and Data Networks.*
16. *Broadband Emergency Communications Systems.*
17. *Prompt, Reliable Traveler Information Systems.*
18. *Partnerships with News Media and Information Providers.*

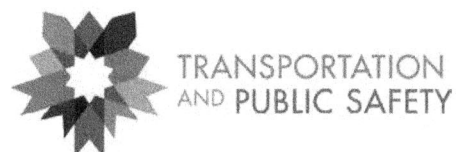

- ❀ Promoting multi-disciplinary discussion on the **long-term vision of effective and efficient TIM Programs**;

- ❀ Addressing **TIM as an institutionalized and sustainable program** that is viewed as a core public safety mission;

- ❀ **Integrating transportation as a full public safety partner**;

- ❀ **Collectively discussing TIM core concepts**, including protecting the lives of responders and motorists, reducing congestion and fuel consumption, enhancing the livability of communities, and improving the environment; and

- ❀ **Ensuring safe, effective and efficient response** to highway and traffic incidents while enhancing transportation emergency preparedness, through:

  - **Legislative Action** – Identifying opportunities to influence State and local legislative action that would clarify and strengthen current TIM statutes (i.e., Move Over and Quick Clearance laws).

  - **Policy Development** – Promoting performance measures, clearance policies, and setting a national research agenda.

  - **Training** – Incorporating TIM and responder safety into existing discipline training at the State, regional and local levels, including full national deployment of SHRP 2 TIM Responder Training course and train the trainer program.

  - **National Outreach** – Engaging the insurance and towing industries, partnering with freight community, and involving the public in reducing fatalities among public safety, transportation, and towing and recovery personnel.

Participants represented transportation and public safety agencies and professional organizations throughout the country. The participants were recognized leaders in their respective fields, representing the agencies listed on the following page. A full list of participants is available in Appendix A – Summit Participants.

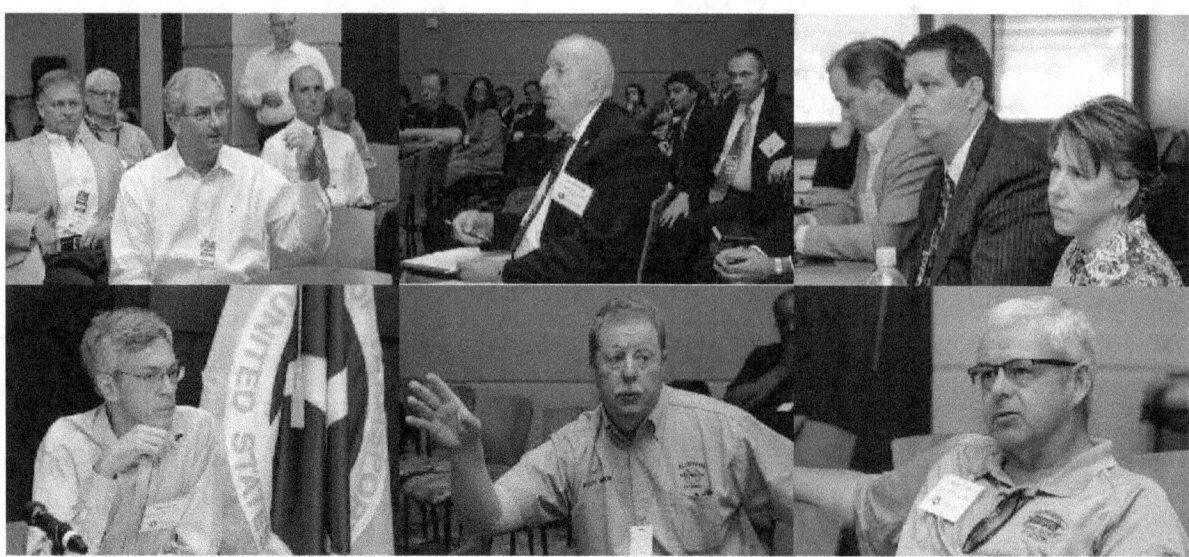

Figure 3: Summit participants from law enforcement, fire, emergency medical services, and transportation agencies discuss opportunities to improve the state of the practice in traffic incident management.

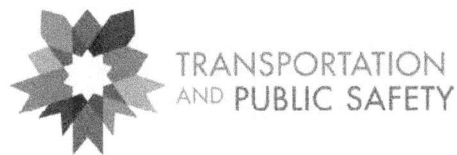
TRANSPORTATION
AND PUBLIC SAFETY

Organizations Represented:

- *American Association of State Highway and Transportation Officials*
- *Arizona Department of Transportation*
- *Arizona Highway Patrol*
- *California Highway Patrol*
- *Champaign, Illinois Fire Department*
- *City of Schertz, Texas*
- *Cumberland Valley Volunteer Firemen's Association Emergency Responder Safety Institute*
- *Federal Highway Administration*
- *Florida Highway Patrol*
- *International Association of Chiefs of Police*
- *International Association of Fire Chiefs*
- *Louisiana State Police*
- *Michigan Department of Transportation*
- *Minnesota Department of Transportation*
- *Minnesota State Patrol*
- *Montana Highway Patrol*
- *Montana State University, Fire Services Training School*
- *National Association of State EMS Officials*
- *National Traffic Incident Management Coalition*
- *National Volunteer Fire Council*

- *New Hampshire Department of Safety*
- *New York State Department of Transportation*
- *North Carolina Department of Transportation*
- *Ohio Department of Transportation*
- *South Carolina Highway Patrol*
- *South Dakota Highway Patrol*
- *Tennessee Department of Transportation*
- *Tennessee Highway Patrol*
- *Texas Department of Transportation*
- *United States Department of Transportation*
  - *Federal Highway Administration*
  - *Federal Motor Carrier Safety Administration*
  - *National Highway Traffic Safety Administration*
  - *Office of the Secretary of Transportation*
  - *Research and Innovative Technology Administration*
- *United States Fire Administration*
- *University of Maryland*
- *Washington State Patrol*
- *White House Office of Intergovernmental Affairs*
- *Wisconsin Department of Transportation*

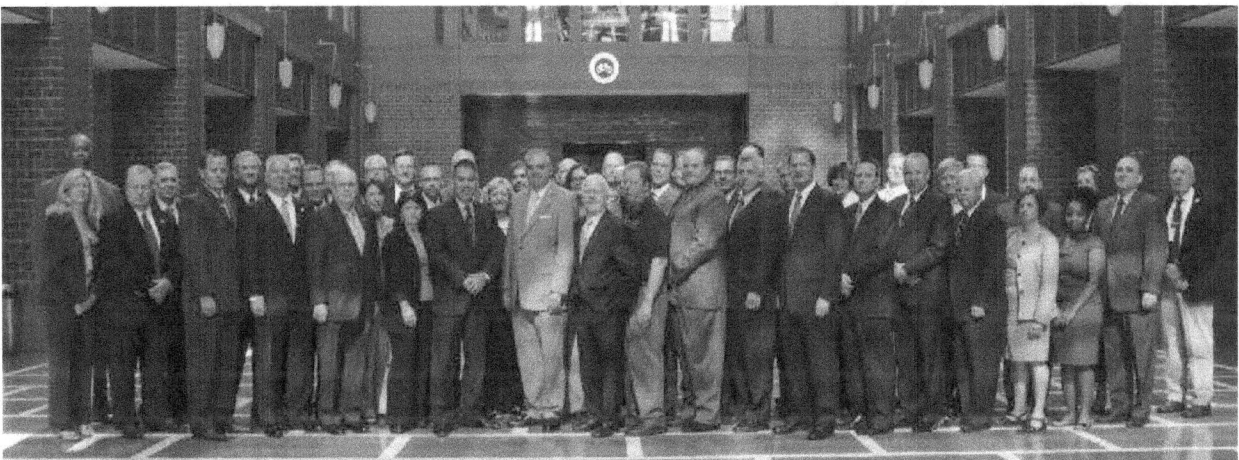

Figure 4: Summit attendees with Secretary of Transportation Ray LaHood, June 26, 2012

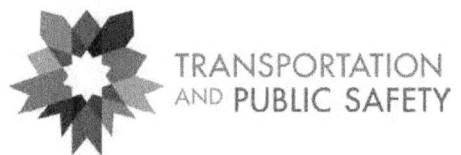
TRANSPORTATION AND PUBLIC SAFETY

Following Posting of the Colors by the United States Capitol Police, Secretary of Transportation Ray LaHood welcomed the participants to the Summit. In his remarks, Secretary LaHood thanked participants for their contributions to the safety of the Nation's roadways. The Secretary discussed successes in safety that have contributed to the recent decline in the number and rate of fatalities. He attributed these successes to effective laws, rigorous enforcement, the dedication of public agencies, and collaborative partnerships. Secretary LaHood thanked all attendees for their participation in the summit and their commitment to public safety, and concluded by sharing his belief that the Nation cannot afford to compromise on safety.

Greg Nadeau, Deputy Administrator for FHWA, also welcomed the group and expressed his appreciation for participants' work in keeping the Nation's transportation system safe and operational through effective enforcement and emergency response. He appealed to participants to support and endorse FHWA's SHRP 2 TIM Responder Training, noting that this vital initiative, among other legislative, policy, training, and outreach activities, will contribute to a culture of improved interagency communication and coordination. Deputy Administrator Nadeau reiterated FHWA's commitment to reducing line-of-duty deaths and injuries among emergency responders and highway workers, as well as mitigating the hazards, delays, and economic and environmental impacts caused by traffic incidents and secondary crashes.

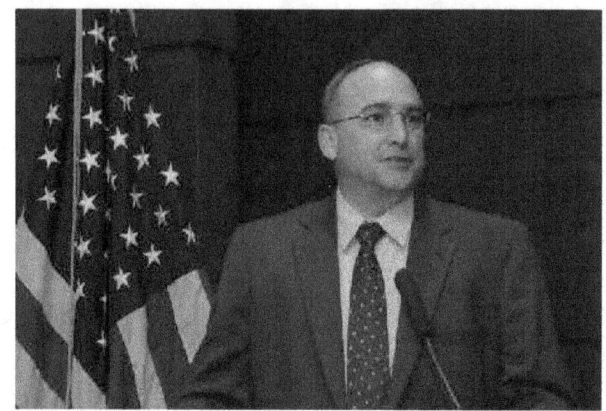
Figure 5: FHWA Deputy Administrator Greg Nadeau addresses Summit participants.

Jeff Paniati, Executive Director of FHWA, reinforced remarks made by Deputy Administrator Nadeau and Secretary LaHood. He was impressed with the progress that has been made in building relationships between the law enforcement, fire, emergency medical services, and transportation disciplines to advance TIM goals. Executive Director Paniati characterized TIM as a vital tool to improving public safety and mobility, but emphasized the need to make it a routine part of transportation and public safety agency operations through clear legislation, policies for quick clearance and TIM performance measurement, multi-disciplinary training, and effective outreach. He committed FHWA to playing a leadership role in developing and advocating for TIM solutions, but asked for participants' support and input in identifying the most pressing issues and needs. Mr. Paniati suggested that this unified effort will contribute to safer roads and an improved ability to move people and goods.

II. TIM State of the Practice

Overview

Most participants attending the Summit believed that partnerships among law enforcement, fire, emergency medical services, and transportation agencies have grown stronger in deploying TIM strategies. The creation of numerous State and regional TIM coalitions and programs, as well as NTIMC, signals a shift toward collaborative emergency response and incident management. However, there was consensus that there is room for improvement in leveraging TIM principles to improve safety and mobility. TIM also presents opportunities to address funding challenges through partnerships and more efficient use of staff.

The following sections detail sessions that addressed policy, legislation, training, and outreach strategies. Participants discussed innovative solutions for enhancing TIM strategies, policies, and procedures, as well as the effectiveness of legislation on safe, quick clearance. Discussions also focused on education and outreach to TIM practitioners and drivers to ensure maximum public and responder safety and compliance with Move Over, Driver Removal, and Quick Clearance laws.

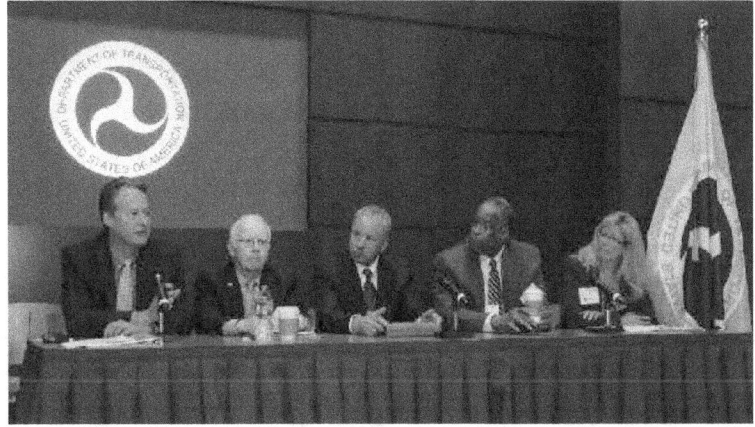

Figure 6: (From left to right) Jeff Paniati (FHWA), Tony Kane (AASHTO), Chief Hank Clemmenson (IAFC), Chief John Batiste (IACP/Washington State Patrol), and Heather Schafer (NVFC) discuss opportunities to advance Traffic Incident Management

Policy

Performance Measurement

While TIM practices can improve roadway safety and congestion, agencies can only determine the extent of this impact through performance measurement. Measuring performance in responding to and clearing incidents is a powerful tool in tailoring policies and training for maximum benefit. Improvements in response and clearance times reinforce the benefit of collecting TIM performance measures throughout the agency and to transportation and public safety partners.

Captain Jeff King and Lieutenant Colonel James McGuffin of the Arizona Department of Public Safety discussed the use of TIM performance measures in Arizona. In particular, Arizona has used performance metrics focused on roadway and incident clearance times and secondary crashes as it broadens its TIM approach to address all incidents, rather than just major incidents. The focus of their TIM efforts had traditionally been aimed at medium and large incidents, which typically garnered media attention and generated greater traffic congestion and complaints. In many cases, these incidents were actually secondary collisions, which originated from a smaller primary incident such as a minor crash or even a traffic stop. Collecting performance measures on all traffic incidents, large and small, has prompted the Department of Public Safety to shift their focus from a few major incidents that occur several times per month

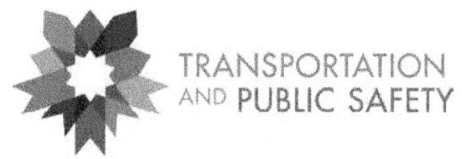

to smaller incidents that occur several times per day. This shift in focus can dramatically increase the overall benefits of TIM.

While the impacts of minor incidents are not as significant individually as those of major incidents, collectively they represent serious potential for safety concerns and delays. In 2011, over seventy percent of Arizona's crashes were minor in nature, resulting in damage to property only. Even though the overall duration of these incidents was lower, their frequency compared to major incidents creates far more cumulative delay and risk for secondary collisions and responder injuries and deaths. During Arizona's initial implementation of its revised TIM strategy between 2010 and 2011, the Department of Public Safety saw a much larger overall reduction in incident clearance times on minor incidents (property damage only) compared to major incidents in the Phoenix metropolitan area (see Figure 8). This dramatic reduction highlights the possibilities for improving responder safety at the national level using simple, effective performance measures.

Reductions in roadway and incident clearance times represent only a portion of the total benefit. Effective TIM practices also reduce the hazards associated with distraction caused by primary incidents. For every minute that these distractions remain on the roadway, the average risk of a secondary collision increases by 2.8 percent[1]. Put another way, on average one secondary collision occurs every 35 minutes that the primary incident remains unresolved. Therefore, even small reductions in incident clearance times can drastically reduce the risk of a secondary incident. Finally, the time savings that Arizona has been able to demonstrate frees up responders and highway workers to perform other activities.

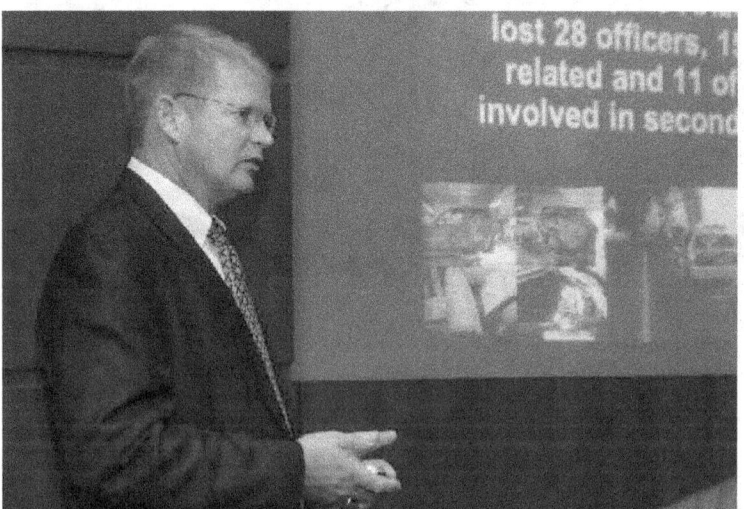

Figure 7: Captain Jeff King, of the Arizona Department of Public Safety, discusses the agency's implementation of TIM performance measures

---

[1] M. Karlaftis et al., *ITS Impacts on Safety and Traffic Management: An Investigation of Secondary Crash Causes,* ITS Journal, Vol. 5, pp. 39-52

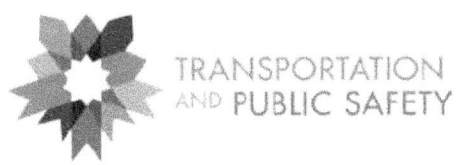

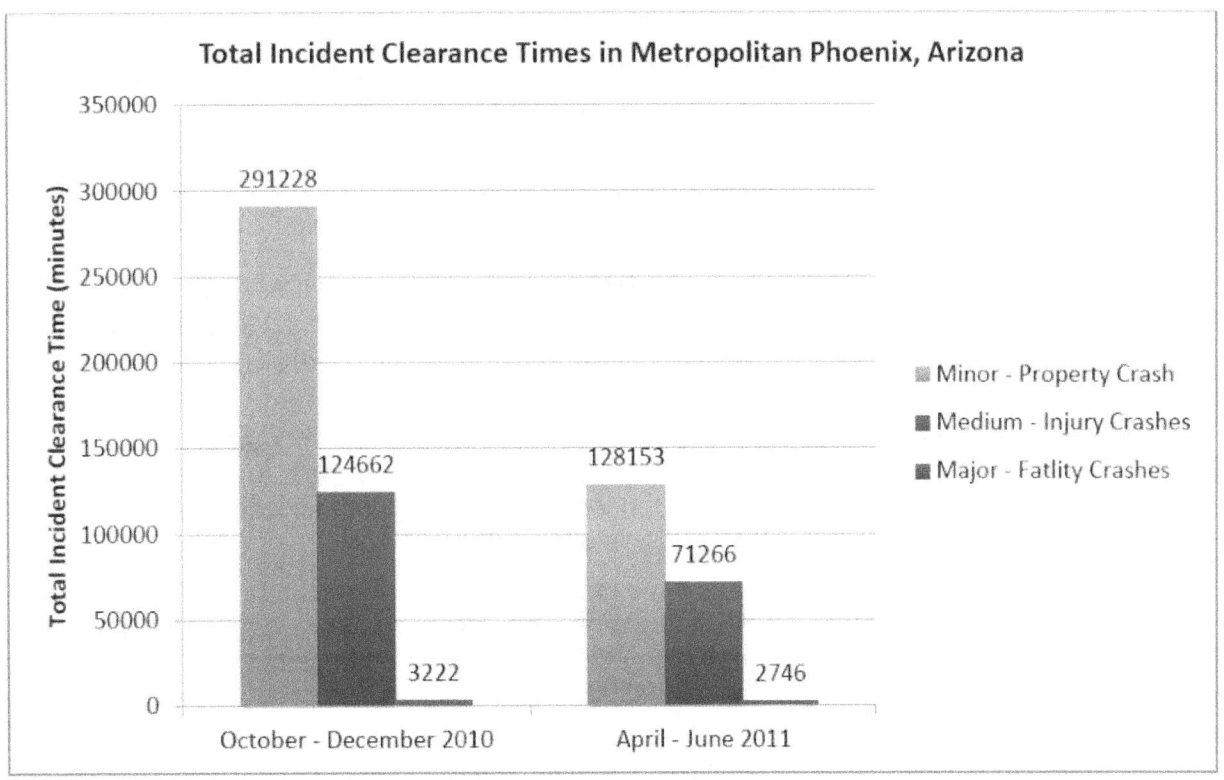

Total Incident Clearance Times in Metropolitan Phoenix, Arizona

Legend:
- Minor - Property Crash
- Medium - Injury Crashes
- Major - Fatlity Crashes

Y-axis: Total Incident Clearance Time (minutes)

October - December 2010: 291228, 124662, 3222

April - June 2011: 128153, 71266, 2746

Figure 8: Changes in Phoenix area incident clearance times associated with Arizona's application of TIM to minor incidents (Source: Arizona Department of Public Safety)

Managing Complicated Mobility and Safety Data

Measuring performance and improving TIM procedures requires robust data that are easily accessible and comprehensible. Incident response involves a variety of agencies representing diverse disciplines, so relevant data are typically stored in multiple databases in separate jurisdictions. Michael Pack of the University of Maryland Center for Advanced Transportation Technology Laboratory offered an example of a comprehensive system for accessing and analyzing transportation operations and incident response data. This Regional Integrated Transportation Information System (RITIS) combines traffic, event, parking, weather, signal, computer-aided dispatch, and transit data for the Washington, D.C. metropolitan area. RITIS offers users access to both real-time data and analysis tools, as well as tools to explore archived data. Integrated and accessible data systems, as demonstrated by Mr. Pack, represent potentially powerful tools for the incident response community to work smarter and faster. Graphics and analysis that used to take dedicated researchers months to prepare can now be developed quickly by any responder agency staff in order to convey the value

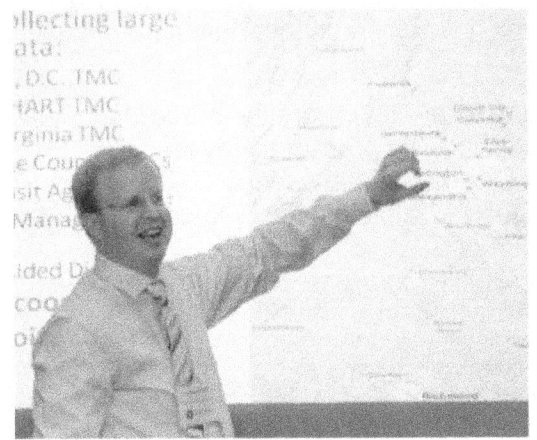

Figure 9: Michael Pack, Director of the University of Maryland Center for Advanced Transportation Technology Laboratory, demonstrates the capabilities of RITIS

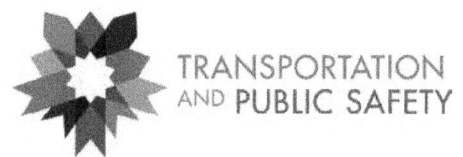TRANSPORTATION
AND PUBLIC SAFETY

of their programs to decision makers and to the public.

Other Innovative Policy Approaches

Chief John Batiste of the Washington State Patrol (WSP) described several of his agency's innovative approaches to improving incident management:

- **Instant Tow Dispatch Protocol** – WSP uses Washington State Department of Transportation (WSDOT) cameras to monitor traffic conditions, identifying any incidents that require towing assistance. Previously, a tow truck operator would not be dispatched until a trooper arrived at the scene of the incident and determined the need for towing assistance. Now, when WSP identifies an incident using the cameras, it dispatches WSP troopers and a tow truck operator simultaneously. This change resulted in significant reductions in delay, in part, because the tow truck no longer is caught in traffic while responding to the incident.

- **Incident Response Program** – WSDOT's Incident Response Program deploys trained maintenance workers on major routes to aid stranded drivers and clear minor incidents. The availability of these WSDOT responders to address minor incidents allows WSP troopers to focus more on major incidents and other law enforcement responsibilities.

- **Major Incident Tow Program** – Washington State's Major Incident Tow Program provides incentives to towing operators who clear major incidents quickly. Under the Program, towing operators who respond to incidents involving tractor-trailer combinations, busses, or trucks over 40,000 Gross Vehicle Weight, qualify for a $2,500 bonus if they can clear the incident within ninety minutes.

- **Critical Reviews** – WSP conducts post-incident reviews with partner agencies following any incident response that exceeds ninety minutes to understand and address the factors that increase incident clearance times. WSP reports the results of these reviews to the Governor, who uses the CompStat approach, first introduced by the New York City Police Department, to oversee critical statewide issues.

In light of increased constraints on resources, participants also discussed the use of partnerships with the private sector to improve incident response. Some States have partnered with private sector insurance companies to provide incident response services similar to Washington State's Incident Response Program. Some transportation-related businesses, such as auto insurers, sponsor roving driver assistance vans along major corridors during peak travel times.

Finally, participants discussed the importance of State and local TIM programs in advancing the state of incident management. While informal, agency-specific TIM practices may lead to improvements in safety and clearance times, formal, documented, multi-agency TIM programs can leverage the benefits these individual practices and lead to sustainable deployment of TIM strategies.

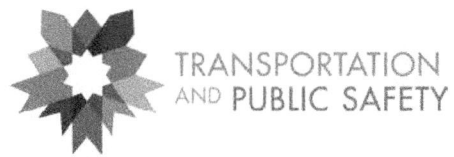

Legislation

Move Over Laws

As of July 2012, every State has adopted a Move Over law, requiring drivers to change lanes or reduce speed when approaching a stopped emergency vehicle. Chief Grady Carrick of the Florida Highway Patrol discussed research results on compliance with Florida's Move Over law and the effects of different emergency lighting configurations. His study, conducted with the University of Florida, found generally high levels of compliance with the lane-change provision of the law but substantially lower compliance among drivers who chose to slow down instead. However, many drivers who changed lanes did not have a sufficiently large gap to maintain a safe distance from other vehicles. The study also found that drivers were more likely to comply with the law when blue and red emergency lights were activated, as opposed to amber arrows that Florida Highway Patrol also installs in its vehicles.

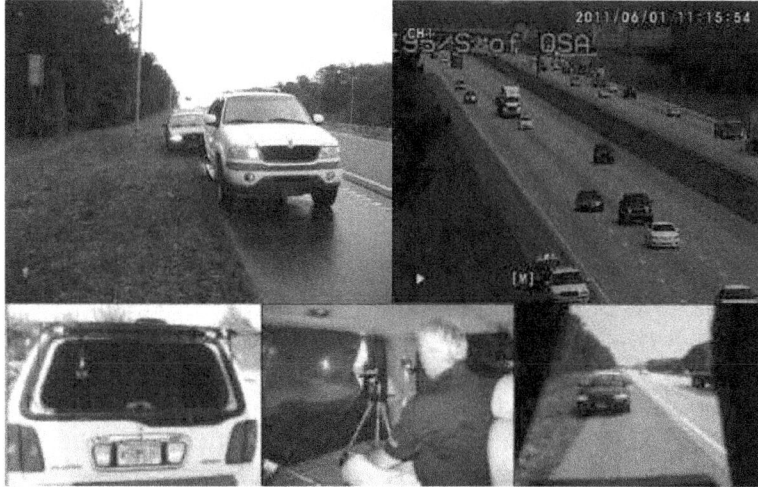

Figure 10: In a study on compliance with Move Over laws' and the effects of emergency lighting on compliance, the Florida Highway Patrol placed a patrol car and research vehicle at the roadside to simulate a traffic stop and recorded the speed and lane behavior of passing vehicles (Photos: *Florida Highway Patrol and Florida Department of Transportation*).

Based on his research, Chief Carrick suggested changes to public messaging of Move Over laws (Section III contains additional discussion on outreach related to Move Over laws) as well as additional research on the effects of Move Over laws in congested areas and outcomes associated with Move Over laws.

Training

SHRP 2 National TIM Responder Training

Congress authorized SHRP 2 as part of the Safe Accountable Flexible Efficient Transportation Equity Act: A Legacy for Users (SAFETEA-LU) to provide funding to TRB to research better ways to improve the safety, renewal, reliability, and capacity of the Nation's highway system. In pursuit of these goals, the SHRP2 partner organizations – TRB, AASHTO and FHWA – recognized the need for a multi-disciplinary training course that provides responders with a shared understanding of requirements and responsibilities for incident management. TRB led the development and pilot testing of a live multi-disciplinary training course and corresponding train-the-trainer course to address the need for coordinated incident response. TRB is in the process of transferring responsibility to FHWA for deploying both courses.

The training course is designed to be taught modularly in about ten hours, in an environment that includes responders from multiple communities – namely, fire, law enforcement, emergency medical services, and transportation. The course includes classroom sessions, a tabletop exercise in which responders must assume an unfamiliar role (e.g., a police officer could play

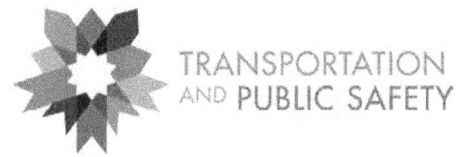

the role of a firefighter), and a practical exercise that allows students to practice various scenarios and become familiar with the equipment available through the different responder groups.

FHWA has established a goal of conducting between fifty and seventy train-the-trainer sessions over the next two to three years in order to prepare 1,000 to 1,500 trainers. FHWA has set an ambitious target for these trainers to reach over one million responders over the next ten years with the multi-disciplinary training course. In order to reach this goal, TRB is currently developing an online version of the course, which should be ready for implementation in fall 2013.

Outreach

History of National TIM Promotion

FHWA Office of Transportation Operations Director Mark Kehrli and Wisconsin DOT Director of Traffic Operations and NTIMC Chair John Corbin each recounted the efforts that have raised the national profile of integrated incident management. FHWA first released its *Traffic Incident Management Handbook* in 1991 to promote practices, tools, and technologies for advancing the state of incident management. FHWA also worked with the American Trucking Associations Foundation in the early 1990s to conduct a series of twenty outreach conferences around the country to build consensus for coordinated incident response. AASHTO, FHWA, the Intelligent Transportation Society of America, and TRB convened TIM practitioners and policy experts in 2002 to identify opportunities to improve TIM practices. This National Conference on Traffic Incident Management highlighted the importance of multidisciplinary, executive dialogue in improving the state of the practice and in influencing action at the local level.

National TIM Coalition

NTIMC launched in 2004 following the National Conference on Traffic Incident Management. It was designed to be a forum in which the public safety and transportation communities could share information about effective practices and coordinate TIM strategies at the national level. That year, NTIMC members participated in an international scan on TIM practices in Europe, during which it learned that TIM is a national policy issue for European countries, where compliance with best practice is strongly encouraged. Following this scan, NTIMC ratified the National Unified Goal in 2007, focusing national attention on the importance of TIM to addressing safety and congestion issues in the United States.

NTIMC continues to promote the National Unified Goal and work with the transportation and public safety communities to standardize TIM best practices. NTIMC enables a national network of TIM programs at the State, regional, and local levels.

TIM Network

In order to more broadly involve the responder community in TIM outreach and implementation of the National Unified Goal, NTIMC established the TIM Network in 2009. The TIM Network seeks to supplement the benefits of training by continually sharing information and best practices with its members on a real-time basis.

The TIM Network currently reaches 1,400 members in 44 States through messaging that resounds with these passionate and enthusiastic TIM practitioners. Through its website (www.timnetwork.org), Facebook page, and Twitter account, the TIM Network shares timely information about incidents involving emergency responders and offers forums in which its members can hold national, multi-disciplinary dialogues every day.

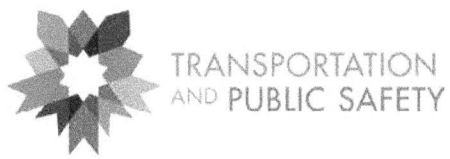

FHWA has conducted a TIM self-assessment of States, regions, and localities since 2003, but revised it in 2007 to more closely align with the National Unified Goal. The self-assessment now covers three main areas: Strategic (organization of and institutional support for TIM program); Tactical (policies and procedures used by field personnel); and Support (tools and technologies that support TIM).

Scores in each area have improved over a baseline representing responses from the 2003-2005 assessments; the average score overall in 2011 was 42 percent higher than the baseline. Mark Kehrli suggested that these scores signal increased attention on the importance of TIM by leaders in transportation and public safety agencies, but cautioned that sustaining this trend will require a sustained effort to institutionalize support for TIM programs.

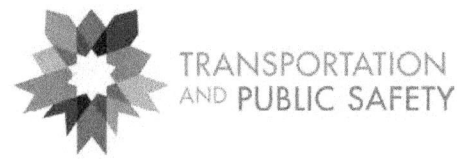
TRANSPORTATION
AND PUBLIC SAFETY

III. Challenges and Opportunities in Enhancing TIM Nationally

Throughout the Summit, participants discussed challenges and opportunities in enhancing or implementing effective TIM programs, procedures, and legislation. The following sections summarize the most prominent issues identified by participants.

Coordination

Challenge – Responder groups do not have a history of coordination

Incident responders have traditionally focused on specific agency responsibilities as they manage and clear incident scenes. Each responding agency or group has a different mission but they share common goals and priorities – safe, efficient, and effective incident management. Participants described instances in which critical tasks have been carried out sequentially and separately, whereas coordination between responder groups would have resulted in faster clearance times and safer incident sites. Moreover, this lack of coordination occasionally results in conflict or confusion over roles, leading to unnecessary and traffic delays.

Opportunity – Regular coordination can improve incident response, save time and lives

Coordination and the elimination of institutional barriers lie at the core of TIM programs and practices. Participants urged better coordination among responder communities at all levels of government. TIM executive leadership meetings can allow agency leaders to discuss issues of national significance, while State, regional, and local TIM coordination meetings are vital to assuring the most efficient and effective response to traffic incidents. Regular communication and coordination enables each responder group to understand the responsibilities and priorities of their partners and provides opportunities to identify procedures that can save time and improve safety.

Institutionalization and Sustainability

Challenge – Institutionalization encourages cooperation

Successful TIM practices require collaboration and coordination among a diverse group of responders in a highly stressful, fluid environment. These responders must be able to communicate and work closely together under extreme time pressures toward a common set of goals while reporting to different agencies with different priorities. Deploying a successful TIM program will enhance on-scene activities but requires that each agency involved is committed and will ensure that their staff participates meaningfully in the process.

Opportunity – Leadership can empower responders

Policies to promote TIM may document the supported practices of an agency, but participants suggested that documentation does not necessarily lead to institutionalization. Instead, they believed that commitment to these practices and principles by leaders can empower responders to implement them on a routine basis. For example, involvement of responder agency leaders in multi-disciplinary groups (i.e., regional, State, and national TIM coalitions) will resonate with working level personnel. Furthermore, participants described instances in which direct communication from leadership was necessary to ensure that new policies were followed. For example, when one State law enforcement agency instituted a policy allowing officers to use newly installed push-bumpers to move disabled vehicles to a safe refuge, few officers followed the procedures initially. Officers only began to use the policy once agency leadership briefed

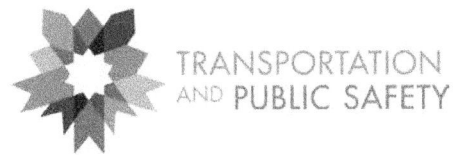

them directly and assured them that the safety and congestion benefits of this policy were worth the potential for minor damage to the disabled vehicles.

Challenge – Champions are vital, but long-term viability transcends individuals

Many summit presenters and participants attributed success in TIM practices and procedures to specific individuals in leadership positions. While acknowledged as an important component of institutionalizing TIM practices, participants agreed that TIM programs need to look beyond individual champions to ensure sustainability. Relying on dedicated leaders can lead to a TIM program that dissolves or loses momentum once key individuals leave an agency. As a result, participants agreed that agencies need to consider sustainability from the outset by identifying how TIM programs will transcend individuals.

Opportunity – Document, review, and revise TIM procedures; Measure performance to maintain momentum

Participants agreed that agencies need to institutionalize TIM practices in order to ensure their long-term sustainability. New procedures or changes to existing TIM procedures should be documented in formal policies and agreements between agencies. Furthermore, regular meetings between disciplines can reinforce these procedures and provide opportunities to identify and address concerns.

At the State, regional, and local levels, the use of performance measures can also keep agencies working towards a common set of goals through changes in leadership. Consistently applied metrics not only push an organization to continually improve, but also allow it to demonstrate the effectiveness of programs to new administrations.

Participants also suggested that an executive group composed of leaders from the public safety and transportation communities can guide national progress toward sustainable TIM practices at the national level. This group can help guide the long-term implementation of the SHRP 2 responder training as well as disseminate and promote the use of innovative TIM practices.

Consistency

Challenge – Move over or slow down?

Though every State has passed a Move Over law, the specifics of these laws vary and are not always clear to the public. Some Move Over laws apply to all stopped vehicles at the roadside with warning lights activated, including civilian vehicles with four-way flashing lights, highway maintenance vehicles, and emergency vehicles with strobe lights, while others are limited to emergency vehicles. Furthermore, Move Over laws vary in their required actions for passing drivers; drivers may comply with most Move Over laws by decreasing their speed instead of changing lanes but the required speed drops are not consistent between States. For instance, Georgia requires drivers to "reduce the speed of the motor vehicle to a reasonable and proper speed for the existing road and traffic conditions" while neighboring Florida requires drivers to reduce their speed to twenty miles per hour below the posted speed limit.

Opportunity – Promote (but don't mandate) consistency

Participants discussed the merits of a model Move Over law to ensure nationwide consistency, but agreed that the laws should remain statewide in nature. However, they suggested that USDOT can play a role in disseminating research and best practices on Move Over law implementation and public awareness campaigns.

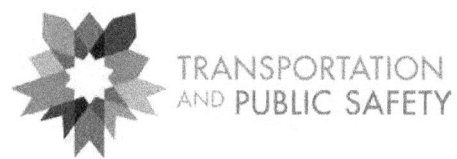

Public Awareness

Challenge – TIM and responder safety laws cannot be effective without public awareness

About half of States have enacted laws requiring drivers to remove their vehicle from travel lanes if involved in a minor, non-injury incident (Driver Removal laws). However, participants suggested that these laws are not well understood by the public, in some cases to such an extent that drivers are reluctant to move vehicles until the arrival of a law enforcement officer, even when the law requires them to do so. Such reluctance does not arise from disagreement with the law, but rather a lack of familiarity with it and a fear of penalties from moving a vehicle from a crash scene[2].

Similarly, the public may be unfamiliar with how to comply with Move Over laws. Drivers unaware of their option to slow down may instead opt to merge into a gap of insufficient size, introducing unnecessary risk to other drivers.

Opportunity – Changing driver behavior takes time, but can be achieved through effective marketing and education

Participants agreed that additional marketing and outreach is needed in States with Driver Removal and Move Over laws. Variable message signs, billboards, and media partnerships can spread the message to the public. States should also take advantage of driver education and licensing procedures to educate drivers on their responsibilities under these laws by including their requirements in new driver education courses and materials.

Participants suggested that the messaging for general education and outreach on these laws should focus on their benefits to individual drivers. Driver Removal laws, when followed, can mitigate excessive congestion from minor incidents and prevent non-injury crashes from escalating into severe or fatal secondary crashes.

Quick Clearance Education

Challenge – Ingrained practices conflict with new quick clearance procedures

States often face opposition to laws and policies that conflict with previous practices or are perceived to interfere with stakeholder interests. For instance, most States that have enacted Driver Removal laws also have quick clearance policies or legislation that allow law enforcement, transportation, and other public agencies to remove disabled vehicles or hazardous cargo from travel lanes, even without the consent of the owner. Some responders are reluctant to follow these procedures for fear of damaging vehicles, while insurers may also oppose these practices for the same reason. Other quick clearance policies can conflict with previous practices and challenge long-held beliefs about incident response. For example, where previous procedures suggest that all lanes of a road should be closed to clear an incident, newer quick clearance practices designate procedures for safely clearing an incident while leaving one or more lanes open to travel.

Opportunity – Educate relevant communities about the benefits of quick clearance

Participants agreed that additional education and outreach is needed to promote the use of existing quick clearance legislation, policies, and procedures. Responders in States with

---

[2] In certain cases, especially with commercial vehicles, insurers prohibit drivers from moving vehicles involved in an incident until an insurance recovery crew arrives. Washington State maintains legislation that protects commercial vehicle operators from penalties associated with moving their vehicles from minor incident scenes.

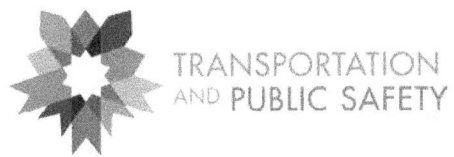

Authority Removal laws should receive education on appropriate conduct under the law as well as assurance that decisions in accordance with such laws will not be punished. Furthermore, States and FHWA should educate insurance providers on the benefits of Driver Removal and Authority Removal legislation. While these practices may cause minor damage to disabled vehicles, their mitigating effect on congestion and secondary crash risks surely prevents more serious damage to vehicles and drivers. Participants suggested that FHWA can promote the benefits of quick clearance nationally through an education, outreach, and public relations toolkit and example legislation.

Conflicting Priorities

Challenge – Different priorities, common goals

Participants acknowledged that the priorities of different responder groups have impeded success in practicing collaborative incident management. Each responder group – transportation, law enforcement, fire and rescue, emergency medical response, and towing – arrives at the scene of a crash with a different immediate objective. Law enforcement personnel need to manage traffic around the scene of a crash while also documenting the circumstances and issuing citations or making arrests, when necessary. Fire and emergency medical services (EMS) personnel are typically focused solely on controlling hazards and ensuring that crash victims receive medical attention. Transportation personnel are responsible for informing other drivers of the incident, providing alternate route information, and clearing debris from the roadway. Participants offered an example of how these differing priorities have resulted in conflict at a crash scene in which fire personnel prefer that all lanes of traffic be blocked while law enforcement and transportation personnel are concerned about causing excessive backups when a partial road closure could ensure an adequate level of safety for crash victims and responders.

Opportunity – Competition to collaboration

Each responder community needs to be aware of and understand the priorities of other responders. Furthermore, responders need to recognize how the priorities and actions of each group contribute to common goals: the safety of responders and the public. Emergency personnel who block access to all travel lanes may not be aware that the additional congestion increases the risk of a secondary crash. Conversely, first responders may not recognize all of the hazards of a particular crash scene.

Considering the needs of the towing industry will also contribute to more successful incident response. Participants cited instances where responders requested the wrong type of towing equipment to clear a crash, leading to additional delays while the tower dispatched different equipment. Instead, participants recommended policies requiring responders to describe the scene to a tow dispatcher but precluding them from requesting specific equipment, leaving it to the towing company to determine which equipment is needed.

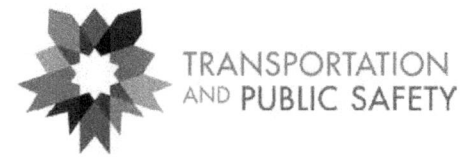
TRANSPORTATION
AND PUBLIC SAFETY

IV.   Recommendations

National Leadership and Legislation

Throughout the Summit, participants discussed the benefits and challenges associated with TIM and quick clearance legislation and policies. Driver Removal, Move Over, and Authority Removal laws can drastically reduce exposure of responders and drivers to secondary crashes but they can only be effective if there is widespread awareness and compliance. Participants recommended the following considerations and actions in order to increase the effectiveness of TIM legislation:

Recommendations: National Leadership & Legislation (NLL)	
Action #	Action Item
NLL-1	Define & Develop Model TIM Safe, Quick Clearance Legislation for consistency & wider adoption
NLL-2	Conduct Additional Research on Compliance with Move Over Laws
NLL-3.1	Establish Structure to Advance Post-Summit Action Items Recommended to FHWA
NLL-3.1	Establish National TIM Executive Leadership Group for policy issues & needs
NLL-3.2	Establish National TIM Technical Working Group
NLL-3.3	Establish National Networking Group to aid in outreach

- ❂ *Define Model TIM Legislation* – Move Over laws, in particular, lack consistency among States. While generally similar, laws differ in their requirements for slowing down and in their definitions of emergency vehicles. Summit participants considered the notion of a national Move Over law, but they ultimately decided that this would be infeasible. However, the development of model legislation could guide States to adopt laws that are more consistent. More broadly, model States could be identified to contribute to the development of a TIM best practices toolkit.

- ❂ *Conduct Additional Research on Compliance with Move Over Laws* – Participants suggested that additional research is needed on the effects of emergency lighting on Move Over compliance in order to issue guidance to law enforcement agencies.

- ❂ *Executive Leadership Group* – National, executive-level attention on TIM is vital to maintaining a sense of strategic priority. The creation of a national TIM leadership group will provide a forum for State and Federal agencies to discuss timely issues and maintain accountability on progress towards national goals. Summit participants discussed the need for executive leadership on TIM and recommended the following structure:

  - – *Executive Working Group* – A relatively small, executive group will include membership from the key organizations that represent TIM practitioners. Each organization will nominate a primary and alternate representative based on their position in order to ensure full representation at each meeting and maintain consistency in the event of staff turnover. Participants suggested that the Executive Working Group include committee leaders from vital organizations (including the State and Provincial Division and Highway Safety Committee of IACP and the Safety, Health, and Survival and EMS Sections of IAFC) as well as executive leadership of these organizations, though the latter may be invited as "non-voting" members. This group will meet up to twice per year to discuss TIM issues of national

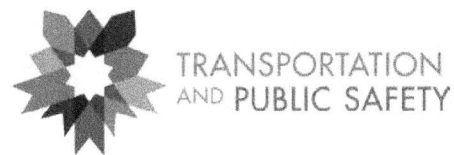

significance and identify barriers to, and opportunities to promote, progress towards national goals. Participants suggested that the Executive Working group may replace the role of NTIMC, as it relates to developing national strategies to advance TIM.

Current NTIMC members may be asked to join either the Executive Working Group or the Technical Working Group. In addition to convening the Executive Working Group, FHWA will also provide administrative support.

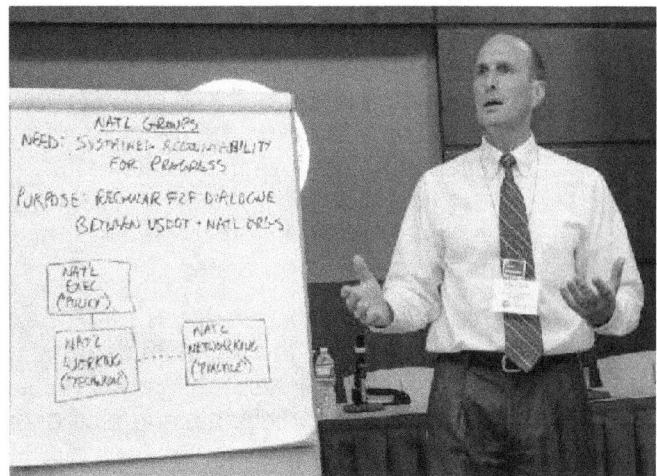

Figure 11: John Corbin, State Traffic Engineer for the Wisconsin Department of Transportation, discusses the proposed structure of a TIM Executive Working Group, Technical Working Group, and National Networking Group

- *Technical Working Group* – A Technical Working Group that involves a broader set of stakeholders will act in an advisory capacity for the Executive Working Group. The Technical Working Group will develop recommendations for the Executive Working Group's consideration and will also be responsible for acting as an intermediary between the Executive Working Group and the responder communities.

- *National Networking Group* – A National Networking Group should be established in parallel with the Executive Working Group and Technical Working Group as a forum for TIM practitioners to share information on the state of the practice. This National Networking Group could include opportunities for virtual and in-person exchange of ideas among TIM responders and will be formed using the TIM Network as a basis.

TIM Institutional and Sustainability Actions

Institutionalization and Sustainability

Throughout the Summit, participants emphasized the need to institutionalize TIM practices and procedures and foster sustainable TIM programs. Participants proposed the following recommendations for FHWA to pursue in order to advance institutionalization of TIM:

- ❖ *Encourage major metropolitan areas to develop TIM committees as a platform for discussing differing goals and interests.*

- ❖ *National Sharing of Knowledge and Experiences* – Collect and share noteworthy practices on how TIM committees and leadership can empower TIM practitioners.

TIM Performance Measurement

Discussions at the Summit highlighted the importance of TIM performance measures in justifying and continually improving TIM programs, legislation, and policies. Participants recommended that the following issues be considered in deploying TIM performance measures:

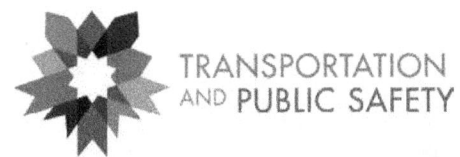
❖ **Develop a Consistent Definition of a Secondary Crash** – Capturing occurrences of secondary crashes on incident report forms is a key requirement for establishing TIM performance measures. However, before this can occur, consensus needs to be reached at the State level, and ideally at the national level, on the definition of a secondary crash. Uniform criteria for reporting secondary crashes will allow consistent comparisons of performance measures between States.

❖ **Begin with High-Priority, High-Volume Routes** – Given the potential demand on resources of collecting data and measuring performance, participants suggested that States begin by focusing on their highest-priority roads, such as Interstates or other major National Highway System roads. TIM has the greatest potential to improve incident clearance times and resulting backups on highly-travelled roads, so performance measures beginning in these areas will be most useful to agencies in refining TIM practices and highlighting success.

❖ **Educate Responders on the Importance of Performance Measures** – Buy-in from responders who are ultimately responsible for collecting performance data is critical. Responders need to be consulted on the feasibility of collecting performance data. Furthermore, responders who do not understand the importance of the data they are expected to collect may negatively impact data quality, completeness, and accuracy. Conversely, responders who recognize the value of performance data will be more likely to approach the task as a core responsibility, rather than a collateral duty. Messaging that emphasizes the relationship between performance measures and personnel safety will be most effective in conveying this value.

Recommendations: Institutional & Sustainability (I&S)	
Action #	**Action Item**
I&S--1	Encourage major metro areas to develop TIM Committees as a platform to discuss differing goals & interests
I&S--2	Collect and share good practices on how TIM Committees & leadership can empower the TIM Practitioners
I&S--3	Adopt TIM Performance Measurement (PM) Systems to Determine Response and Program Effectiveness
I&S--3.1	Develop a National, Consistent Definition of a Secondary Crash, Place on Crash/Incident Intake Forms & Collect data
I&S--3.2	Encourage States to Begin Collecting Incident-Specific Performance Measurements with High-Priority, High-Volume Routes
I&S--3.3	Educate TIM Responders on the Importance of Collecting & Reporting Performance Measures
I&S--3.4	Encourage States to Gather Additional TIM PM Data on Struck-By Incidents
I&S--3.5	Establish National TIM PM Pilots in Selected Jurisdictions

❖ **Perfection is Ideal, But Not Required** – While any agency's ultimate goal should be high-quality, complete, and accurate data, participants acknowledged that this may not be immediately feasible for many agencies due to funding constraints. They suggested that data that are not perfect should not prevent a State from measuring its performance.

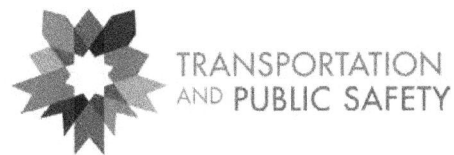

❦ ***Additional Data on Struck-By Incidents Puts the Problem in Context*** – In addition to collecting data on clearance times, participants identified a significant need for better data on the number of responders and vehicles that are involved in both fatal and non-fatal secondary crashes. While data on fatal secondary incidents are more robust, participants suggested that injury and property damage data could be nearly as valuable in improving and building support for TIM programs. Such data would not only highlight the safety impacts of these crashes on responders, but also the direct cost to agencies in terms of medical leave and replacing equipment.

❦ ***TIM Performance Measurement Pilot*** - FHWA recommended the establishment of a TIM Performance Measurement Pilot. Jurisdictions participating in the pilot would work in a cooperative effort with the Arizona Department of Public Safety, which currently collects the following TIM performance measures:

– *Roadway Clearance Time* – The time interval between the first recordable awareness of an incident (detection, notification, or verification) by a responding agency and first confirmation that all traffic lanes are open to traffic;

– *Incident Clearance Time* – The time between the first recordable awareness of the incident and the time at which the last responder has left the scene; and

– *Secondary Crashes* – The number of incidents that occur within the incident scene or within the queue, including the opposite direction resulting from the original incident, after the time of detection of the primary incident.

Professional Capacity Building

FHWA will rely heavily on the support of national organizations and State, regional, and local agencies as it deploys the SHRP 2 National Traffic Incident Management Responder Training course and train-the-trainer session. Though TRB and FHWA have conducted several pilot implementations of the course and have funding to provide trainers for a few sessions per State, it will depend on trainers from the transportation and public safety communities to deliver the course and ultimately reach FHWA's aggressive targets. Participants discussed FHWA's implementation of the SHRP 2 National TIM Responder Training course and other potential professional capacity building efforts, and recommended the following strategies:

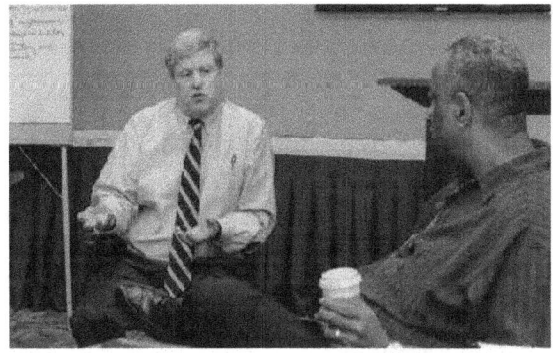

Figure 12: Paul Jodoin, from the FHWA Office of Operations, discusses implementation of the National TIM Responder Training with Chief John Batiste and other Summit participants.

❦ ***Perform Additional Outreach and Education for Responders*** – Participants discussed issues where responders are not familiar with their responsibilities under TIM legislation. Participants reported instances where responders are hesitant to remove disabled vehicles using push-bumpers for fear of punishment if they cause additional damage. Participants recommended that nationally applicable outreach and education materials are needed to increase awareness of TIM legislation requirements.

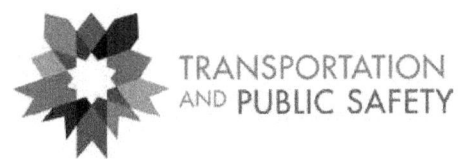

❖ **Convey Importance through USDOT Leadership Endorsement** – Participants recommended that Secretary of Transportation LaHood send a formal letter to leaders in State transportation and public safety agencies emphasizing the importance of the National TIM Responder Training course to:

– Maintaining the safety of emergency responders;

– Quickly reaching, treating, and transporting crash victims; and

– Efficiently and effectively clearing incidents to avoid congestion.

The Secretary's letter should underscore the message that FHWA's preferred configuration for the training is live with representation from multiple disciplines, though the agency recognizes that local staffing and other resource limitations may limit certain agencies to the use of an online training format instead. Trainers should be encouraged to have multiple representatives from each responder discipline at each live training session.

❖ **Executive Briefings/State Transportation and Public Safety Summits** – Once State leaders receive a letter from Secretary LaHood, participants recommended that FHWA Division Administrators, in coordination with State DOT, State Police, and Fire leadership, invite representatives from each responder discipline to attend a State transportation and public safety summit. During this summit, FHWA and State transportation and public safety leadership can brief key staff about the importance and benefits of the training. Endorsement by senior officials in State law enforcement, fire, and EMS communities will significantly promote interest among responders.

These events can also be used to discuss State-specific implementation approaches for the training. Participants advised FHWA that not every State, region, or locality is at the same level of maturity or readiness for the training. For some, the training will reinforce existing knowledge and skills while others will be exposed to entirely new concepts during the training.

Recommendations: Professional Capacity Building (PCB)	
Action #	Action Item
PCB--1	Perform Additional Outreach & Education for Responders
PCB—2	Convey Importance of National-Provided TIM Responder training through USDOT Leadership Endorsement
PCB—3	Conduct Executive Briefings/State Transportation and Public Safety Summits on the Need for Training
PCB—4	Develop & Implement Full Range of Training Courses
PCB-4.1	Develop & Conduct SHRP2 TIM Responder Training Course
PCB-4.2	Develop & Conduct TIM Advanced Workshops
PCB-4.3	Develop & Conduct TIM Executive Leadership Awareness Training
PCB—5	Market the Training Outcomes
PCB—6	Explore Possibility of Continuing Education Credits
PCB—7	Pursue Opportunities for Earlier Availability of Online Training
PCB—8	Leverage Multi-Disciplinary Partnerships

❖ **Develop and Implement a Full Range of Training Courses** – FHWA, in collaboration with multi-disciplinary experts in the field of TIM, identified several gaps in training practitioners and managers in TIM operations and program administration. As a result,

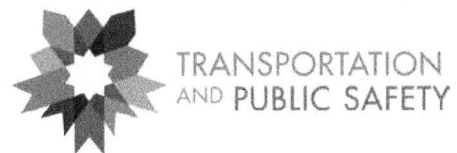
several courses must be developed for implementation by State and local TIM practitioners, particularly in the fields of transportation, law enforcement, and fire and rescue. These courses would include basic and advanced courses for field personnel, managers, and community planners, as well as individualized training. The participants endorsed the current training under development and encouraged addressing other existing training gaps. Summit participants suggested the following actions by FHWA:

– **Develop and Conduct SHRP 2 National TIM Responder Training Course** – The National TIM Responder Training course was developed through the second Strategic Highway Research Program and presents a unified, multi-disciplinary approach based on new multi-agency standards and best practices. The curriculum has been extensively peer-reviewed and pilot tested in States across the country. SHRP2 is a national partnership of FHWA, AASHTO, and TRB. SHRP2 Solutions is delivering products to enhance the productivity, boost the efficiency, increase the safety, and improve the reliability of the Nation's highway system. Summit participants encouraged FHWA to deploy the SHRP 2 TIM responder training to State and local instructors in the transportation, law enforcement, fire, towing and recovery, EMS, public works and other stakeholder disciplines with the hope that consistent, basic training will develop capacity over the Nation and yield hundreds of thousands trained in good practices and operations over the next three years.

– **Develop and Conduct TIM Advanced Workshops for Mid-Level Managers and Practitioners** – Summit participants encouraged FHWA to continue providing advanced workshops to other metropolitan areas and to expand training to the rural jurisdictions and corridors.

– **Develop and Conduct TIM Executive Leadership Awareness Training** – Summit participants agreed that the leadership training conducted by FHWA with mid-level managers has yielded great success and resulted in increased understanding and support by TIM practitioner supervisors and executives. They encouraged FHWA to continue this process and to provide tools that they may use to brief their own supervisors on the benefits of TIM.

❖ **Market the Training Outcomes** – Summit participants discussed potential strategies for marketing the SHRP2 National TIM Responder Training course to its target audiences. Ultimately, they suggested that the responder communities are most likely to react to the intended outcomes and benefits of the training, specifically responder safety, rapid treatment and transport of crash victims, and efficient incident clearance. Once agencies understand these aspects of the training, they will become more interested in the training content.

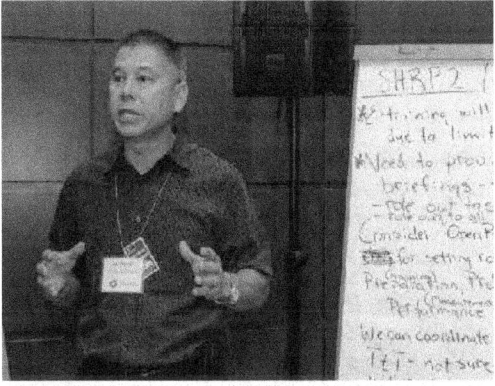

Figure 13: California Highway Patrol Commissioner Joe Farrow discusses recommendations for implementing the SHRP2 National TIM Responder Training course and train-the-trainer session

❖ **Continuing Education Credits** – Participants suggested that offering continuing education

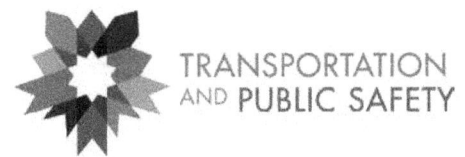
TRANSPORTATION
AND PUBLIC SAFETY

credits in exchange for taking the course would significantly increase interest among responders. The opportunity to earn EMS credits may be particularly appealing to fire personnel, because they are often required but difficult to attain.

- ❋ *Online Training Will Be Vital* – Though TRB and FHWA would prefer that the training be delivered entirely to a live audience, they recognize that this would be infeasible in many situations. Therefore, TRB is currently developing an online version of the training, which participants supported, especially for training responders in rural agencies.

- ❋ *Leverage Multi-Disciplinary Partnerships* – Given the training's multi-disciplinary emphasis, participants recommended that FHWA conduct outreach through multi-disciplinary venues. In particular, they suggested that State emergency managers already interact with all of the TIM disciplines on a regular basis and would therefore be an ideal conduit to responders. Participants also believed that outreach between disciplines would be an effective tactic (e.g., if the head of a State Fire Chiefs Association were to discuss the importance of the training at a regional AASHTO meeting).

Public Awareness and Education

Summit participants reinforced a recurring theme among TIM practitioners: the public is not only not practicing safe operations when involved in an incident, but are often unaware of State and local Safe, Quick Clearance laws, including Move Over and Driver Removal laws or policies. As a result, the group provided a list of recommendations based on this observation:

Recommendations: Public Awareness & Education (PAE)	
Action #	**Action Item**
PAE-1	Conduct Effective Public Awareness Campaign on Safe, Quick Clearance
PAE-2	Perform Additional Outreach and Education for the Public
PAE-3	Deploy Education materials to Communities to Change Behaviors & Educate Public on the Benefits of Safe, Quick Clearance

- ❋ *Conduct Effective Public Awareness Campaign on Safe, Quick Clearance* – Education and outreach campaigns should be deployed to promote the use and benefits of, and compliance with, existing quick clearance legislation, policies, and procedures. Agencies that operate under Authority Removal laws should educate their personnel on what constitutes appropriate conduct under the law and should provide assurance that decisions in accordance with such laws will not be punished. States and FHWA should also conduct outreach to insurance providers to explain and demonstrate the benefits of Driver Removal and Authority Removal legislation. While these practices may cause minor damage to disabled vehicles, their mitigating effect on congestion and secondary crash risks surely prevents more serious damage to vehicles and drivers.

- ❋ *Perform Additional Outreach and Education for the Public* - Participants discussed issues where drivers are not familiar with their responsibilities under TIM legislation. Drivers may be unsure about how to comply with Move Over laws or that moving their vehicle from the scene of a minor incident is not only allowed, but required by Driver Removal laws. Participants recommended that nationally-applicable outreach and education materials are needed to increase awareness of TIM legislation requirements. Messages about complying with Move Over and Driver Removal laws should also be

25

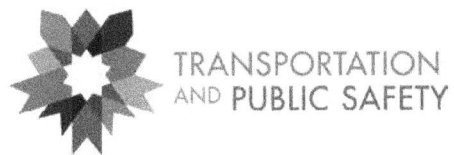
displayed on variable message signs and billboards, and should be included in driver education courses and materials.

- ✿ ***Deploy Educational Materials to Communities to Change Behaviors and Educate the Public on Safe, Quick Clearance*** – Participants suggested that FHWA can promote the benefits of safe, quick clearance nationally by disseminating its Traffic Incident Management Outreach Toolkit (available at <u>ops.fhwa.dot.gov/eto_tim_pse/timtoolbox/</u>) and developing sample legislation, as discussed above in ***National Leadership and Legislation***. Moreover, since changing behaviors starts with youth, driver education curricula around the Nation should emphasize the laws and policies of that State and local jurisdictions. FHWA's TIM Outreach Toolkit includes a template for developing training materials for the classroom and questions for the Department of Motor Vehicles tests.

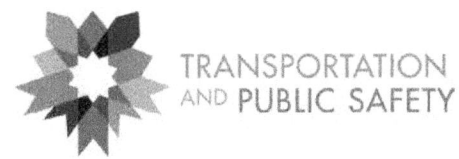
TRANSPORTATION
AND PUBLIC SAFETY

V.   Vision for the Future and Next Steps

National Executive Leadership in TIM

Based on recommendations from the Summit, FHWA will convene an Executive Working Group by the end of the year to hold more in-depth conversations about critical TIM issues in advancing the strategies of the National Unified Goal. In preparation for a meeting of this group, FHWA will identify critical, immediate issues where policy or guidance is needed. These emphasis areas will drive decision-oriented discussions at Working Group meetings and will motivate individual organizations to commit to regular representation on, and participation in, the Working Group. FHWA will set a date for the Group's first meeting that falls before the end of the calendar year.

In its role as a collective of national TIM leadership, the Executive Working Group can serve as a conduit for outreach to nationally significant, non-traditional partner organizations, including the National Governors Association and the National Conference of State Legislatures.

A Trained Community of Responders

FHWA expects its deployment of the SHRP 2 TIM responder training to provide a significant portion of the responder community with a common set of knowledge and skills in traffic incident response and a shared understanding of each other's responsibilities. Within the next two years, FHWA intends to prepare close to 1,300 trainers who will, in turn, deliver the classroom training to more than 90,000 responders. In total, FHWA plans to enable more than 3,000 instructors within the next five years to train close to 325,000 responders. FHWA anticipates that an online version of the course, due in 2013, will reach an additional 1.2 million responders. In total, FHWA's five-year goal represents about two thirds of all emergency responders and highway operations workers in the United States[3]. Full deployment of the National TIM Responder Training will represent a significant step towards realizing the National Unified Goal.

TIM Performance Measurement, Data Collection, and Assessment

FHWA supports the collection and analysis of TIM Performance Measures. FHWA intends to use TIM performance measures to determine the impact of TIM practices and policies on operations and safety, more specifically on reducing responder fatalities and injuries and improving mobility. Using the experience shared by the Arizona Department of Public Safety's Lieutenant Colonel James McGuffin and Captain Jeff King as a basis, FHWA plans to develop a pilot program for collecting TIM performance data and demonstrating safety and mobility benefits.

Reduce Responder and Transportation Personnel Fatalities

Many States have adopted a long-term goal of zero traffic fatalities. While recent trends have been encouraging – there were more than 10,000 or nearly 25 percent fewer fatalities in 2010

---

[3] The Bureau of Labor Statistics estimates that there were approximately 143,000 highway maintenance workers (http://www.bls.gov/oes/current/oes474051.htm), 794,000 sworn law enforcement positions (http://www.bls.gov/ooh/Protective-Service/Police-and-detectives.htm) and 226,000 emergency medical technician and paramedic positions (http://www.bls.gov/ooh/Healthcare/EMTs-and-paramedics.htm) in 2010. The National Fire Prevention Association estimates that there were approximately 1.1 million career and volunteer firefighters in 2010 (http://www.nfpa.org/assets/files//PDF/OS.FDProfile.pdf).

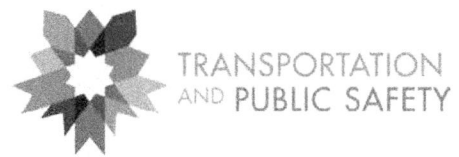

compared to 2005 – preventing roadway fatalities altogether will be a substantial challenge. However, drastically reducing roadway fatalities among emergency responders and highway workers represents a feasible starting point. Effective legislation, policy, outreach, and education strategies can each make significant contributions to reducing responder fatalities, while national TIM leadership can ensure accountability towards responder fatality goals.

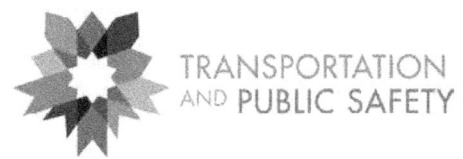
TRANSPORTATION AND PUBLIC SAFETY

VI.   Appendix A – Summit Participants

David Agnew, Director
White House Office of Intergovernmental Affairs

Richard J. Ashton, Grant/Technical Management Manager
International Association of Chiefs of Police

Bernie Arseneau, Deputy Commissioner/Chief Engineer
Minnesota Department of Transportation

Steve Austin, Project Manager
Cumberland Valley Volunteer Firemen's Association Emergency Responder Safety Institute

John Batiste, Chief
Washington State Patrol

Jan Brown, Director of Field Services – South
Federal Highway Administration

Grady Carrick, Chief
Florida Highway Patrol

Hank Clemmensen, Fire Chief
International Association of Fire Chiefs

John Corbin, State Traffic Engineer
Wisconsin Department of Transportation

David Covington, Fire Chief
City of Schertz, Texas

Kevin Daly, Colonel
Minnesota State Patrol

Paul Degges, Chief Engineer
Tennessee Department of Transportation
paul.degges@tn.gov

Linda Dodge, Chief of Staff/Program Manager for Public Safety and Rural Programs
USDOT, Research and Innovative Technology Administration, Intelligent Transportation Systems Joint Program Office

Mike Edmonson, Colonel, Superintendent
Louisiana State Police

Joe Farrow, Commissioner
California Highway Patrol

Mike Flynn, Assistant Director for Field Operations
Ohio Department of Transportation

Tony Furst, Associate Administrator for Safety
Federal Highway Administration

Dia Gainor, Executive Director
National Association of State Emergency Medical Service Officials

Paul Jodoin, Transportation Specialist, Emergency Transportation Operations Team
Federal Highway Administration

Gregory Johnson, Chief Operations Officer
Michigan Department of Transportation

Tony Kane, Director of Engineering and Technical Services
American Association of State Highway and Transportation Officials

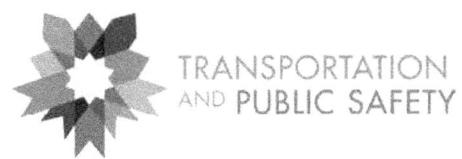
TRANSPORTATION AND PUBLIC SAFETY

Mark Kehrli, Director, Office of Transportation Operations
Federal Highway Administration

Jeff King, Captain
Arizona Department of Public Safety, Highway Patrol Division

Martin Knopp, Division Administrator, Florida
Federal Highway Administration

Tim Lane, Public Safety Liaison
Federal Highway Administration

Ray LaHood, Secretary
United States Department of Transportation

Jeff Lindley, Associate Administrator for Operations
Federal Highway Administration

James McGuffin, Lieutenant Colonel
Arizona Department of Public Safety, Highway Patrol Division

Jeff Michael
National Highway Traffic Safety Administration

Mary Beth Michos, Fire Chief
International Association of Fire Chiefs

Gummada Murthy
American Association of State Highway and Transportation Officials

Greg Nadeau, Deputy Administrator
Federal Highway Administration

T.J. Nedrow
National Volunteer Fire Council

Michael Oliver, Colonel
South Carolina Highway Patrol

Michael Pack, Director
University of Maryland Center for Advanced Transportation Technology

Craig Price, Superintendent
South Dakota Highway Patrol

Carol Rawson, Director of Traffic Operations Division
Texas Department of Transportation
Carol.Rawson@txdot.gov

Eric Rensel
National Traffic Incident Management Coalition, TIM Network

Heather Schafer, Director
National Volunteer Fire Council

Rod Sechrist, Assistant Commissioner for Operations and Asset Management
New York Department of Transportation

Noah Smith, Program Analyst
National Highway Traffic Safety Administration

Earl Sweeney, Assistant Commissioner
New Hampshire Department of Safety

Michael Tooley, Colonel
Montana Highway Patrol

Jennifer Toth, Chief Engineer
Arizona Department of Transportation

Tracy Trott, Colonel
Tennessee Highway Patrol,
Tracy.Trott@tn.gov

Bill Troup
United States Fire Administration
Bill.Troup@dhs.gov

Mike Wagers, Director
International Association of Chiefs of Police, Division of State and Provincial

TRANSPORTATION
AND PUBLIC SAFETY

Butch Weedon
Montana State University, Fire Services
Training School

Keith Williams
Federal Highway Administration

**Jack Van Steenburg, Chief Safety Officer
and Assistant Administrator**
Federal Motor Carrier Safety Administration

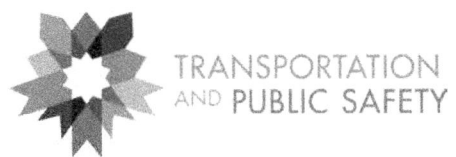

VII. Appendix B – Summit Agenda

Tuesday, June 26, 2012		
8:45am	Posting of Colors Opening Remarks	U.S. Capitol Police Ray LaHood, Secretary, U.S. Department of Transportation
9:10	Welcome	Greg Nadeau, Deputy Administrator, FHWA
9:30	Overview of the Summit	Mark Kehrli, Director, Office of Transportation Operations, FHWA
9:40	Leadership, Innovation and Key Partnership: Advancing Traffic Incident Management for the Future	Panelists: Jeff Paniati, Executive Director, FHWA Tony Kane, Director of Engineering and Technical Services, AASHTO Chief John Batiste, IACP/S&P Chief Hank Clemmensen, IAFC Heather Schafer, Executive Director, NVFC Moderator: Luisa Paiewonsky, Volpe Center
10:45	*Break*	
11:00	Advancing Operations: National Program Overview	Jeff Lindley, Associate Administrator for Operations,

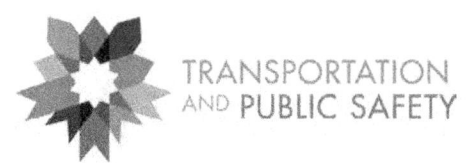

		FHWA
11:30	*Lunch*	*Speaker: David Agnew, White House Director, Intergovernmental Affairs*
1:00	Policy Strategies • Visualizing Performance: Making Sense of Complicated Mobility and Safety Data for Responders and the Public • Reducing Secondary Crashes – Importance of Performance Measures • TIM Performance Measures Pilot Program	Michael Pack, Director, Center for Advanced Transportation Technology, University of Maryland Jeff King, Captain, Arizona Department of Public Safety James McGuffin, Colonel, Arizona Department of Public Safety
2:30	Legislative Strategies • Florida Move Over Law and Effects of Emergency Lighting	Grady Carrick, Chief, Florida Highway Patrol
3:15	*Break*	
3:30	Training Strategies • National TIM Training Initiatives	Paul Jodoin, TIM Program Manager, FHWA
4:00	Outreach Strategies • National Outreach Initiatives • Maximizing Executive Leadership Working Towards Innovative Solutions to Transportation Challenges	John Corbin, Director of Traffic Operations, Wisconsin DOT Mark Kehrli, Director, Office of Transportation Operations, FHWA
5:15	Review of Day 2	Luisa Paiewonsky, Volpe Center

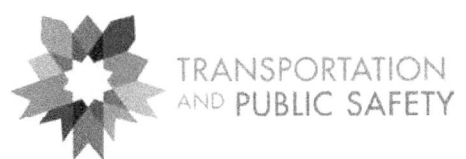
TRANSPORTATION
AND PUBLIC SAFETY

5:30	Adjourn	
Wednesday, June 27, 2012		
8:45am	Overview of Day 2	Luisa Paiewonsky, Volpe Center
9:00	Action Planning – Part A (Breakout Groups)	Facilitators: Cassandra Allwell, Volpe Center Paul Jodoin, Office of Transportation Operations, FHWA Luisa Paiewonsky, Volpe Center Keith Williams, Office of Safety, FHWA
10:00	Small Group Report Out and Discussion	Groups 1 and 2 Designated Spokespersons
10:45	Break	
11:00	Action Planning – Part B (Breakout Groups)	
12:00	*Lunch*	*Speaker: Tim Lane, Public Safety Liaison Program Manager, FHWA*
1:00	Small Group Report Out and Discussion	Groups 1 and 2 Designated Spokespersons
1:45	Video	
2:15	*Break*	
2:30	Action Planning – Part C (Large Group)	Facilitators: Paul Jodoin, Office of Transportation Operations, FHWA Luisa Paiewonsky, Volpe Center
3:30	Closing Remarks	FHWA
4:00	*Adjourn*	

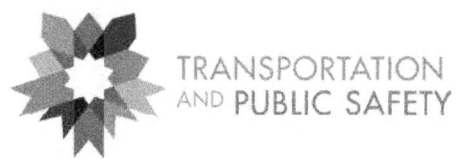

VIII. Appendix C – Summary of Actions

Roadmap for National TIM Leadership & Innovation		
Action #	**Action Item**	**Target Due**
National Leadership & Legislation (NLL)		
NLL–1	Define & Develop Model TIM Safe, Quick Clearance Legislation for consistency & wider adoption	6 to 12 months
NLL–2	Conduct Additional Research on Compliance with Move Over Laws	12 to 18 months
NLL–3	Establish Structure to Advance Post-Summit Action Items Recommended to FHWA	1 to 6 months
NLL–3.1	Establish National TIM Executive Leadership Group (ELG) for policy issues & needs	3 to 6 months
NLL–3.2	Establish National TIM Technical Working Group (TWG)	3 to 6 months
NLL–3.3	Establish National Networking Group to aid in outreach	3 to 6 months
Institutional & Sustainability (I&S)		
I&S–1	Encourage major metro areas to develop TIM Committees as a platform to discuss differing goals & interests	6 to 12 months
I&S–2	Collect and share good practices on how TIM Committees & leadership can empower the TIM Practitioners	6 to 12 months
I&S–3	Adopt TIM Performance Measurement (PM) Systems to Determine Response and Program Effectiveness	18 to 24 months
I&S–3.1	Develop a National, Consistent Definition of a Secondary Crash, Place on Crash/Incident Intake Forms & Collect data	6 to 12 months
I&S–3.2	Encourage States to Begin Collecting Incident-Specific Performance Measurements with High-Priority, High-Volume Routes	12 to 36 months
I&S–3.3	Educate TIM Responders on the Importance of Collecting & Reporting Performance Measures	3 to 18 months
I&S–3.4	Encourage States to Gather Additional TIM PM Data on Struck-By Incidents	3 to 18 months
I&S–3.5	Establish National TIM PM Pilots in Selected Jurisdictions	6 to 18 months
Practitioner Capacity Building (PCB)		
PCB–1	Perform Additional Outreach & Education for the Responders4	1 to 36 months
PCB–2	Convey Importance of National-Provided TIM Responder training through USDOT Leadership Endorsement	1 to 3 months
PCB–3	Conduct Executive Briefings/State Transportation & Public Safety Summits on Training Needs	3 to 18 months

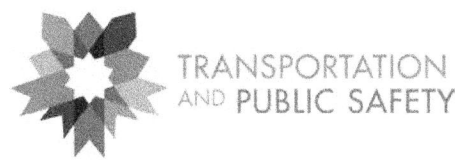

PCB–4	Develop & Implement Full Range of Training Courses	1 to 60 months
PCB–4.1	Develop & Conduct SHRP2 TIM Responder Training Course	1 to 36 months
PCB–4.2	Develop & Conduct TIM Advanced Workshops	1 to 36 months
PCB–4.3	Develop & Conduct TIM Executive Leadership Awareness Training	1 to 36 months
PCB–5	Market the Training Outcomes	6 to 48 months
PCB–6	Explore Possibility of Continuing Education Credits	3 to 18 months
PCB–7	Pursue Opportunities for Earlier Availability of Online Training	3 to 18 months
PCB–8	Leverage Multi-Disciplinary Partnerships	1 to 36 months
Public Awareness & Education (PAE)		
PAE–1	Conduct Effective Public Awareness Campaign on Safe, Quick Clearance	1 to 36 months
PAE–2	Perform Additional Outreach and Education for the Public1	1 to 36 months
PAE–3	Deploy Education materials to Communities to Change Behaviors & Educate Public on the Benefits of Safe, Quick Clearance	1 to 36 months

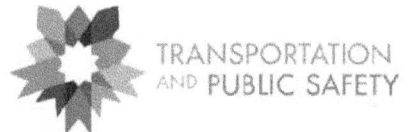
TRANSPORTATION AND PUBLIC SAFETY

Federal Highway Administration

Office of Transportation Operations (HOTO)

1200 New Jersey Avenue, S.E. Washington, DC 20590

FHWA-HOP-12-051